Essential environmental health standards in health care

Edited by John Adams, Jamie Bartram, Yves Chartier

WHO Library Cataloguing-in-Publication Data

World Health Organization.

Essential environmental health standards in health care
Edited by John Adams, Jamie Bartram, Yves Chartier

1.Environmental health — standards. 2.Health-care facilities — standards. 3.Health-care facilities — organization and administration. 4.Health policy. 5.Sanitation — standards. 6.Developing countries. I. Adams, John. II. Bartram, Jamie. III. Chartier, Yves.

ISBN 978 92 4 154723 9   (NLM classification: WX 140)

© World Health Organization 2008

All rights reserved. Publications of the World Health Organization can be obtained from:

WHO Press, World Health Organization
20 Avenue Appia
1211 Geneva 27, Switzerland
Tel: +41 22 791 2476
Fax: +41 22 791 4857
Email: bookorders@who.int

Requests for permission to reproduce or translate WHO publications — whether for sale or for non-commercial distribution — should be addressed to WHO Press at the above address (fax: +41 22 791 4806; e-mail: permissions@who.int).

The designations employed and the presentation of the material in this publication do not imply the expression of any opinion whatsoever on the part of the World Health Organization concerning the legal status of any country, territory, city or area or of its authorities, or concerning the delimitation of its frontiers or boundaries. Dotted lines on maps represent approximate border lines for which there may not yet be full agreement.

The mention of specific companies or of certain manufacturers' products does not imply that they are endorsed or recommended by the World Health Organization in preference to others of a similar nature that are not mentioned.

Errors and omissions excepted, the names of proprietary products are distinguished by initial capital letters. All reasonable precautions have been taken by the World Health Organization to verify the information contained in this publication. However, the published material is being distributed without warranty of any kind, either express or implied. The responsibility for the interpretation and use of the material lies with the reader. In no event shall the World Health Organization be liable for damages arising from its use.

The named authors alone are responsible for the views expressed in this publication.

Printed in India
Designed by Design ONE, Canberra, Australia

The cover photographs are (top to bottom):latrines (World Bank), child washing (World Bank), hospital (Carmem Pessoa-Da-Silva), child drinking (World Bank), woman washing (World Bank), health-care facility (Yves Chartier).

Foreword

Health-care associated infections contribute to morbidity and mortality, and to a loss of health-sector and household resources worldwide. Five to thirty per cent of patients develop one or more infections during a stay in hospital — a significant proportion of which could be avoided. In crises or precarious situations, the number of infections worsens. In some circumstances, people may choose not to seek care because the nearest facilities are not functioning or because treatment is uncertain due to shortages of water, electricity or supplies.

Unsafe health-care settings contribute to a significant proportion of some diseases. Legionellosis is a well-established risk associated with health-care facilities, with an average proportion of health-care associated infections close to 10%. Sharps waste, although produced in small quantities, is highly infectious. Contaminated needles and syringes represent a particular threat because they are sometimes scavenged from waste areas and dump sites, and reused. If poorly managed, they expose health-care workers, waste handlers and the community to infections.

The problem of diseases from unsafe health-care settings is growing worse. Worldwide, there is increasing provision of health care, which is also becoming more complex. Furthermore, an increasing proportion of the population is immunocompromised (and therefore more susceptible to health-care related infection). Without effective action, the situation is likely to deteriorate.

Health-care settings include hospitals, health centres, clinics, dental surgeries and general practitioner facilities. They provide an opportunity to educate visitors and the general population about minimizing disease transmission by providing targeted messages and a "model" safe environment. Messages can also contribute to a safe home environment, which is especially relevant to the trend towards increased home-based care in both developing and developed countries.

The development and implementation of national policies, guidelines on safe practices, training and promotion of effective messages in a context of healthy medical facilities will decrease the number of infections associated with health-care settings.

The international policy environment increasingly reflects the problem of health-care associated infections. The eight United Nations (UN) Millennium Development Goals[1] include goals on maternal health (there are an estimated 529 000 maternal deaths per year), as well as other goals relating to major diseases and infant mortality.

At the same time, the UN Millennium Project[2] and the UN Secretary-General have highlighted the importance of rapidly addressing "quick wins"; that is, identifying specific ways of providing health services to health-care facilities.

Guidelines on environmental health in health care are universally available, but additional guidance for precarious situations is needed.

---

[1] http://www.un.org/millenniumgoals/
[2] http://www.unmillenniumproject.org/

This document deals specifically with essential environmental health standards required for health-care settings in medium- and low-resource countries to:

- assess prevailing situations and plan the improvements that are required
- develop and reach essential safety standards as a first goal
- support the development and application of national policies.

These guidelines have been written for use by health managers and planners, architects, urban planners, water and sanitation staff, clinical and nursing staff, carers and other health-care providers, and health promoters.

Contents

Foreword 3

Acknowledgements 7

Abbreviations and acronyms 9

1 Introduction 11
    1.1 Purpose, scope and audience 11
    1.2 Policy rationale 12
    1.3 Health rationale 13
    1.4 Health-care settings 14
        1.4.1 Large health-care settings 14
        1.4.2 Small health-care settings 14
        1.4.3 Emergency or isolation settings 14
    1.5 Structure 15

2 Implementation 17
    2.1 Positive policy environment 17
    2.2 Steps in managing standards at national, district and local levels 17
    2.3 Roles and responsibilities 19
    2.4 Coordination in the health-care setting 20
    2.5 Using the guidelines to create standards for specific health-care settings 20
    2.6 Assessing and planning minimum standards 20
    2.7 Phased improvements 21
    2.8 Technology choice, operation and maintenance 21
    2.9 Ongoing monitoring, review and correction 22
    2.10 Staff requirements and training 22
    2.11 Hygiene promotion 23

3	Guidelines for setting environmental health standards	25
	3.1 Guidelines and associated information	25
	3.1.1 Guideline structure	25
	3.1.2 Indicators	25
	3.1.3 Guidance notes	25
	3.2 Guidelines	27
4	Assessment checklist	47
5	Glossary	53
6	Further reading	55

Acknowledgements

The World Health Organization (WHO) wishes to express its appreciation to all whose efforts made the production of this document possible. In particular, WHO gratefully acknowledges the contributions of the following experts, who contributed to and reviewed these guidelines.

John Adams
Visiting Lecturer, Liverpool School of Tropical Medicine
Liverpool, United Kingdom

Roger Aertgeerts
Regional Adviser, Water and Sanitation, European Centre for Environment and Health
WHO Regional Office for Europe, Roma, Italy

Sheila Anazonwu
Communications and Development Programme Officer, International Hospital Federation
Ferney Voltaire, France

Jamie Bartram
Coordinator, Programme on Assessing and Managing Environmental Risks to Health
WHO Headquarters, Geneva, Switzerland

Yves Chartier
Public Health Engineer, Programme on Assessing and Managing Environmental Risks to Health
WHO Headquarters, Geneva, Switzerland

Mohd Nasir Hassan
Programme of Environmental Health
WHO Regional Office for Western Pacific, Phnom Penh, Cambodia

Nathalie Isouard
Hygiene hospital technical adviser
Médecins Sans Frontières, Barcelona, Spain

Peter Maes
Coordinator, Department of Water and Sanitation
Médecins Sans Frontières, Brussels, Belgium

Saheen Methar
Head of Academic Unit for Infection Prevention and Control
Tygerberg Hospital & Stellenbosch University, Cape Town, Republic of South Africa

Catherine Noakes
Pathogen Control Research Group, School of Civil Engineering
University of Leeds, Leeds, United Kingdom

Jackie Sims
Technical Officer, Programme on Assessing and Managing Environmental Risks to Health
WHO Headquarters, Geneva, Switzerland

U Kyaw Win
Deputy Director, Environmental Sanitation Division
Department of Health, Yangon, Myanmar

Raki Zgondhi
Urban Health and Environment
WHO Regional Centre for Environmental Health Activities, Amman, Jordan

The development of this publication was made possible with the support and collaboration of the Australian Government's overseas aid programme (AusAID), the United Kingdom Department for International Development, the Swedish International Development Cooperation Agency and the World Patient Safety Alliance.

Abbreviations and acronyms

DPD	N,N-diethyl-p-phenylenediamine
FAO	Food and Agriculture Organization of the United Nations
HBV	hepatitis B virus
HCV	hepatitis C virus
HCS	health care setting
HEV	hepatitis E virus
HIV	human immunodeficiency virus
NTU	nephelometric turbidity units
SARS	severe acute respiratory syndrome
UN	United Nations
WHO	World Health Organization

1 Introduction

1.1 Purpose, scope and audience

Essential environmental health standards in health care contains guidelines for setting standards of safety conditions to provide adequate health care. This document also recommends measures for minimizing the risk of health care-associated diseases for patients, staff and carers.[3]

These guidelines have been written for use by health managers and planners, architects, urban planners, water and sanitation staff, clinical and nursing staff, carers and other health-care providers, and health promoters. They can be used to:

- develop specific national standards that are relevant to various health-care settings in different contexts
- support the application of national standards and set specific targets in health-care settings
- assess the situation regarding environmental health in existing health-care settings to evaluate the extent to which they may fall short of national plans and local targets
- plan and carry out the improvements that are required
- ensure that the construction of new health-care settings is of acceptable quality
- prepare and implement comprehensive and realistic action plans so that acceptable conditions are achieved and maintained.

These guidelines deal specifically with water supply (water quality, quantity and access), excreta disposal, drainage, health-care waste management, cleaning and laundry, food storage and preparation, control of vector-borne disease, building design (including ventilation), construction and management, and hygiene promotion. They are designed primarily for use in health-care settings in precarious situations, and in situations where simple and affordable measures can improve hygiene and health significantly.

In principle, standards are set at the national level and are used at district and local levels to set and work towards specific targets. Therefore, these guidelines provide a basis for setting standards at a national level when this is required; they may be used in a similar way at district and local levels, where appropriate. They are intended to be used, together with existing national standards and guidelines, for creating targets, policies and procedures to be used in each health-care setting. Box 1.1 contains definitions of standards and guidelines.

---

[3] 'Carers' is used in these standards to mean family, friends or voluntary workers who care for a patient at home or who accompany patients to a health-care setting, visit hospitalized patients and provide basic, non-professional care. Carers may be occasional visitors, or they may stay to cook, clean and care for patients in the health-care setting (medical structure or home).

> **Box 1.1 Definitions of standards and guidelines**
>
> **Standards**
>
> Standards are the requirements that must be met to achieve minimum essential environmental health conditions in health-care settings. They must be clear, essential and verifiable statements.
>
> **Guidelines**
>
> Guidelines are the recommended practices to achieve desirable minimum environmental health standards in health-care settings. They are not law, but should be used as guidance.

1.2 Policy rationale

Effective functioning of health-care settings depends on a number of different requirements, including safe and sufficient water, basic sanitation, adequate management of health-care waste, appropriate knowledge and application of hygiene, and adequate ventilation. However, many of these requirements are not available in many health-care settings across the world (WHO, 2004a).

Health-care associated infections affect between 5% and 30% of patients, although the figures could be significantly higher in some contexts (WHO, 2005a). The associated burden of disease is extremely high, is a significant drain on health-sector and household resources, and disproportionately affects vulnerable members of society. Environmental health in health-care settings can significantly decrease the transmission of such infections.

Health-care settings include hospitals, health centres, clinics, health posts, dental surgeries, general practitioner settings and home-based care. Interventions to improve environmental health in health-care settings are intended to reduce the transmission of infections (in health-care settings) and therefore directly reduce the disease burden. They are also targeted at high-risk populations (for example, immunocompromised patients). Health-care settings also provide an educational opportunity to promote safe environments that are relevant to the population at large, and thereby also contribute to safe environments at home and in community settings, such as schools.

The international policy environment increasingly reflects these issues. Among the United Nations (UN) Millennium Development Goals,[4] that is of direct relevance to the goals on improving maternal health (an estimated 529 000 maternal deaths occur per year; WHO 2005c) and reducing child mortality. They also support other goals, especially those on major diseases and infant mortality. The Millennium Project and the UN Secretary-General have also highlighted the importance of rapidly addressing "quick wins" (successful, quick interventions), particularly, providing services to health-care settings and schools (see Box 1.2 below).

Putting policy into practice in this area demands strong links between sectors such as health, water supply and sanitation, planning, building management and construction.

---

[4] http://www.un.org/millenniumgoals/

Box 1.2　UN Millennium Development Goals relating to health-care settings

Goal 4, Target 5 of the UN Millennium Development Goals aims at reducing by two thirds the death rate for children under five.

Goal 5, Target 6 aims at reducing maternal mortality by three quarters.

1.3　Health rationale

Health-care settings are environments with a high prevalence of infectious disease agents. Patients, staff, carers and neighbours of the health-care setting face unacceptable risks of infection if environmental health is inadequate. The health-care setting might even become the epicentre of outbreaks of certain diseases, such as typhus or diarrhoea.

Table 1.1 shows the risks related to environmental health in health-care settings, as well as the main preventive measures that are covered by these guidelines. Some staff may be exposed to radiological or chemical hazards. These require particular preventive measures that are beyond the scope of these guidelines.

Table 1.1　Disease risks and preventive measures in health-care settings

Disease risk	Prevention measures
Airborne infections (e.g. *Legionella*, avian influenza, SARS, tuberculosis)	• Ventilation • Space available per patient • Spacing of beds • Use of separate rooms for highly vulnerable or infectious patients • Use of masks and correct incineration of wastes
Water-, food- or handborne infections (e.g. HEV, diarrhoea)	• Water supply (quality and access) • Excreta disposal • Hygiene facilities • Food hygiene • Hand hygiene
Infection of wounds/surgical incisions from contaminated water, medical devices and dressings (e.g. sepsis)	• Use of single-use medical devices and dressings • Pre-disinfection • Cleaning and sterilization of instruments and dressings • Good-quality water • Asepsis in surgical or dressings procedures
Bloodborne infections due to contaminated needles and syringes, unsafe blood transfusion (e.g. HBV, HCV, HIV)	• Health-care waste management and use of single-use needles and syringes • Safe blood transfusion
Heat- and cold-related stress and discomfort (e.g. higher fever)	• Heating, ventilation, air-conditioning (HVAC) and insulation
Vector-borne disease transmission (e.g. malaria, dengue, leishmaniasis)	• Control of disease vectors in and around buildings • Protection of patients • Protection of infrastructure

HBV, hepatitis B virus; HCV, hepatitis C virus; HEV, hepatitis E virus; HIV, human immunodeficiency virus; SARS, severe acute respiratory syndrome

1.4 Health-care settings

These guidelines are intended for use in precarious health-care settings where simple, robust and affordable solutions to infection control are required. They apply to a range of health-care settings, from home-based care through to district and central hospitals. Three broad types of health-care settings (discussed below) illustrate the issues involved in environmental health:

- large health-care settings providing a range of outpatient and inpatient care
- small health-care settings providing outpatient care and outreach activities
- emergency or isolation settings.

1.4.1 Large health-care settings

Examples of large health-care settings providing a range of outpatient and inpatient care include district hospitals and other referral health facilities. Disease transmission risks are substantial, given the presence of infectious patients and extended contact with other patients, staff and carers. The full range of water supply, sanitation and hygiene facilities and services covered by these guidelines needs to be provided.

Financial and material resources may be scarce, but there is usually a substantial human resources capacity, with medical, nursing, pharmacy and technical services staff potentially able to contribute to infection control.

1.4.2 Small health-care settings

Examples of small health-care settings providing outpatient care and outreach activities include primary health-care centres in rural, periurban and urban areas. As there is normally no inpatient care, disease transmission risks are limited. A more limited range of facilities and services covered by these guidelines needs to be provided and the basic requirements are relatively simple.

Financial and material resources may be scarce and support from the health authorities may be inadequate, particularly in remote rural areas and poor peri-urban areas.

1.4.3 Emergency or isolation settings

Emergency or isolation settings include isolation or treatment facilities for routine emergencies as well as infectious diseases such as cholera, severe acute respiratory syndrome and viral haemorrhagic fever, and therapeutic feeding centres in emergencies. These settings may be stand-alone in crises ("open situations") or set up under tents in refugee camps ("closed situations"); alternatively, they may be attached to, or part of, an existing health-care setting. Disease transmission risks are particularly high in these settings.

Intensive management of water supply, sanitation, hygiene and waste is required to protect staff, carers and patients from diseases such as cholera and viral haemorrhagic fever. Some specific measures may be required that go beyond the scope of these guidelines, and specialized references should be consulted (see the list of "Further reading").

1.5 Structure

These guidelines are organized into four main sections:

- Section 1 provides an overview of the purpose, scope and rationale for the guidelines.
- Section 2 discusses how these guidelines may be used at national, district and local levels, and identifies roles and responsibilities of stakeholders.
- Section 3 contains the 11 guidelines, each of which is accompanied by a set of indicators (measures for whether the guidelines are met) and guidance notes (advice on applying the guidelines and indicators in practice, highlighting the most important aspects that need to be considered when setting priorities for action).
- Section 4 provides a checklist of assessment questions for each of the guidelines presented in Section 3, to measure the extent to which the guidelines are followed and to identify areas for action.

Specific terms are explained in the glossary, and references and further reading are provided in the reference list.

2 Implementation

This section highlights the importance of policy that encourages implementation of these guidelines, and outlines the steps and roles and responsibilities at national, district and local levels. It also provides information on applying the guidelines to specific health-care settings; using them to develop minimum standards (which can be used to assess standards that are already in place); choosing appropriate technology for implementation; and ensuring ongoing monitoring, improvements and staff training.

2.1 Positive policy environment

Positive policies are required at national, state, regional, district and health-setting levels to encourage appropriate levels of environmental health in health-care settings. A supportive policy environment should allow stakeholders at district and health-setting levels to establish effective governance and management arrangements to plan, fund, implement and coordinate improvements and maintain standards, based on these guidelines.

2.2 Steps in managing standards at national, district and local levels

As discussed in Section 1.1, these guidelines can be used to set standards at a national, district or local level. Once standards have been set, there are essential steps for managing them at national, district and local (health-care setting and community). These steps are shown in Table 2.1.

The three levels presented in the table are intended as a general illustration of how related activities are required at different levels. The way in which these activities are organized in any given context will depend on country-specific arrangements but, in principle, standards are set at the national level and are used at district and local levels to set and work towards specific targets.

Intergovernmental organizations, such as the World Health Organization (WHO), and national and international nongovernmental organizations, may play an important role at all levels. This should also be taken into account in each country.

Table 2.1 Steps in establishing and managing appropriate standards at national, district and local levels

	National level	District level	HCS or community level
1	• Review existing national policies and ensure that there is a national policy framework that supports improved conditions in HCSs.	• Raise awareness on environmental health in HCSs among key stakeholders at district level.	• Mobilize support from health workers, local communities and other local stakeholders to achieve and sustain a healthy health-care environment. • Promote a working climate that encourages patient and staff safety.
2	• Ensure that national bodies exist for setting and monitoring standards.	• Ensure that an appropriate body or service exists at district level for overseeing compliance with national standards.	• Create and assign responsibility to a local body to oversee the implementation of national standards at HCS level. • Promote a working climate that encourages patient and staff safety.
3	• Provide national expertise and knowledge through information dissemination mechanisms.	• Provide expertise and resources for assessment and planning at local level.	• Assess existing conditions, consult local stakeholders (including staff and local community) and plan improvements and new developments.
4	• Review national standards and add to them if needed. • Ensure that there is an effective regulatory framework that encourages and supports compliance.	• Ensure that the national regulatory framework is reflected in guidance and support for compliance at district level. • Develop and use guidelines where national standards do not exist.	• Define a set of targets, policies and procedures for implementing national standards and/or guidelines in a way that reflects local conditions. • Define how targets, policies and procedures will be applied.
5	• Provide and/or facilitate funding for national programmes.	• Allocate funding for planned improvements and new developments.	• Seek funding for planned improvements and new developments.
6	• Monitor progress at national level and promote consistent application of standards in all regions and at all levels.	• Ensure oversight of improvements and new developments to ensure the consistent application of national standards in all HCSs.	• Oversee implementation of planned improvements and new developments.
7	• Produce training and information materials appropriate to a range of health-care settings. • Ensure appropriate curriculum for health-care worker training.	• Provide appropriate training and information to health-care workers.	• Provide advice and training to health-care workers and patients.
8	• Periodic review and update of policies, standards, training contents, evaluation and monitoring tools.	• Inform key stakeholders at district level on updated environmental health components in HCSs.	• Mobilize support from health workers, local communities and other local stakeholders to improve, achieve and sustain a healthy health-care environment. • Promote a working climate that encourages patient and staff safety.

HCS, health-care setting

2.3 Roles and responsibilities

Table 2.2 presents the role and responsibilities of stakeholders at district and local levels. It also outlines some of the things they can do to help achieve and maintain adequate environmental health conditions in health-care settings. The list is not exhaustive and can be added to in any particular context.

Table 2.2 Roles and responsibilities for implementing guidelines and standards for environmental health in health-care settings

Stakeholder group	Contribution to improved environmental health in HCSs or home care
Patients	• Comply with procedures for use and care of water and sanitation facilities, and observe appropriate hygiene measures.
Patients' families and carers	• Comply with procedures for use and care of water and sanitation facilities, and observe hygiene measures. • Encourage patients to do the same.
Health-care workers	• Carry out disease prevention duties (such as cleaning, health-care waste management, hand hygiene and asepsis in health care) consistently and well. • Care for and maintain water and sanitation facilities. • Encourage patients and carers to adopt appropriate behaviours. • Participate actively in achieving and maintaining targets.
HCS managers	• Plan and implement programmes to set, achieve, monitor and maintain targets. • Create conditions in which staff are motivated to meet and maintain targets.
Health authorities	• Provide resources and direction for setting, achieving and maintaining targets.
Environmental health services	• May collect and dispose of health-care waste in a centralized facility. • Provide specialist advice for identifying problems and recommending solutions for water supply, sanitation and hygiene.
Education sector	• Raise awareness in medical schools and other sectors. • Provide training for the health sector.
Politicians	• Provide and mobilize political and financial support for improvements.
Public works and/or water and sanitation sector	• Ensure correct design and construction of buildings and sanitary infrastructure and maintain services to HCSs as a priority.
Construction and maintenance industry, including local contractors	• Provide skilled services that comply with national standards for construction, maintenance and repair of buildings and sanitary infrastructure.
National and international Funding bodies	• Provide funding for new HCSs, upgrading or renovation of existing ones and ongoing maintenance of targets.
Other communities	• Participate in disease control sessions through community health organizations that might exist. • Report on health-care waste found outside HCSs.

HCS, health-care setting

The level of participation described above is achievable through the allocation of resources and commitment at all levels.

Effective linkages between different government sectors, and between the public sector, the private sector and local communities, are essential. Local intersectoral bodies, such as village or district development committees, may be useful for joint planning, implementing and monitoring of improvements.

2.4 Coordination in the health-care setting

Managing the various and interdependent aspects of environmental health at the level of the health-care setting should involve all staff, as well as patients and carers (see Section 2.3). There should be a clearly identified body with the authority and resources required to carry out steps 3–7 (in the health-care setting or community level column), in Table 2.1, above.

In hospitals and other larger settings, a committee may be required for planning, coordinating and monitoring implementation of targets. Members of the committee should include managers, clinicians, technical and ancillary staff.

In smaller settings, such as basic health posts, this role may be taken on by one staff member or volunteer, who should receive support from environmental health officers or other infection control staff based at the district level.

In these guidelines, the term "infection control committee" is used to describe a body at the local or health-care setting level. This body might be a committee or a single person, and may be responsible for all aspects of infection control, or may focus more specifically on water supply, sanitation, hygiene, ventilation and health-care waste management.

2.5 Using the guidelines to create standards for specific health-care settings

The guidelines in Section 3 reflect general principles for providing adequate health care and minimizing the health-care associated disease risk to patients, staff and carers. They can be used, as follows, for creating specific targets or standards appropriate for individual health-care settings, or different types of health-care settings:

- **Review the 11 guidelines**, which are narrative statements describing the situation to be aimed for.
- **Identify major areas that require attention in relation to specific guidelines**. Consider on-site conditions that might affect the way that the guidelines are interpreted in practice. Note that on-site constraints, such as lack of funding or lack of a suitable water source, should not be taken into consideration at this stage. The aim is first to define appropriate standards required in a particular setting, then to seek ways to meet those standards, rather than defining limited standards that are insufficient.
- **Use national standards or the indicators under each guideline to define specific targets or standards**, such as the number of users per toilet or the quantity of water per person per day required. The indicators provide benchmarks that reflect current understanding of appropriate levels of service required to create and maintain healthy care environments. The guidance notes provide advice on taking account of local conditions when using the indicators for setting specific targets or standards and on intermediate steps to reaching them.

2.6 Assessing and planning minimum standards

Once specific standards have been defined for a particular health-care setting or type of setting, they can be used as a checklist to determine how and to what extent the existing situation falls short of them. This will identify specific problems that need addressing. See Section 4 for an assessment checklist.

Analysing the reasons for shortfalls, in as inclusive a way as possible, is important because most solutions will require the participation of multiple parties, including patients, carers, health-care workers and health managers. A useful tool for this analysis is the problem–solution tree (see Box 2.1). Objectives should be understandable and motivating to all those concerned by their achievement, and progress towards achieving them should be possible to measure and describe easily and clearly.

Box 2.1   The problem–solution tree

The problem–solution tree is a simple method to identify problems, their causes and effects, and then define objectives for improvement that are achievable and appropriate for the specific conditions of each health-care setting. The problem–solution tree is performed as a group activity through the following steps:

1. Discuss any major aspects of the current situation where water supply, sanitation, health-care waste management and hygiene targets defined for the health-care setting are not met. Write each one in large letters on a small piece of paper (e.g. A6 size) or a postcard.

2. For each major problem, discuss its causes by asking "why?" For each of the contributing problems identified, ask "why?" again, and so on until root causes for each problem have been revealed and agreed. Write all the contributing problems in large letters on a piece of paper or postcard and stick them on a wall, arranged in a way that reflects their relation to each other and to the major problem.

3. For each of the contributing problems noted, discuss possible solutions. Check that these solutions contribute to solving the major problems identified by asking "what?" to identify the effects of the action. Some solutions proposed will probably have to be abandoned because they are not realistic given current conditions, or because they do not have sufficient impact on the major problems.

4. Once a number of feasible solutions have been agreed, they should be phrased as objectives. For each objective, the group can then discuss and agree on a strategy (how the objectives can be reached), responsibilities (who will do what), timing, resources and requirements.

2.7   Phased improvements

Many health-care settings are currently far from achieving acceptable levels of environmental health and may have no suitable facilities at all, because of lack of resources, skills or adequate institutional support. Often, achieving appropriate standards will not be possible in the short term. Therefore, steps should be taken both to prioritize improvements and to work in a phased way so that the most urgent problems can be identified and addressed immediately, and other benefits subsequently achieved. See Box 3.1 in Section 3 for advice on intermediate measures for situations where long-term standards cannot be met rapidly.

2.8   Technology choice, operation and maintenance

Maintenance, repair and eventual replacement of environmental health facilities should be taken into account while they are being designed and built. As far as possible, facilities should be hard-wearing, durable and possible to maintain without specialist skills or equipment. Technology should be chosen taking account of local capacities for maintenance and repair. In some cases, it may be necessary to choose a lower level of service to avoid essential equipment that cannot be repaired when it breaks down. For example, it may be better to keep an open, protected well, rather than equip it with a cover slab and pump, until there is a reliable system in place for maintaining and repairing the pump.

Responsibilities for operation and maintenance should be clearly defined, and appropriate expertise provided (see Section 2.9). Maintaining, repairing and replacing water supplies, sanitation, ventilation systems and health-care waste facilities should be planned and budgeted for from the beginning of a programme to improve health-care settings or build new ones.

2.9 Ongoing monitoring, review and correction

Maintaining acceptable conditions requires ongoing efforts at all levels. The role of the infection control committee in ensuring regular monitoring of environmental health conditions is critical. The local department of environmental health should be a major partner, providing expert monitoring and advice. For example, health-care settings should be included in regular water quality surveillance and control programmes.

A monitoring system should use a limited set of indicators (such as behavioural indication) that are easily and frequently measured to identify problems and correct them in a timely way. For example, water shortages at handwashing points may be monitored by staff according to an organized schedule, and signalled immediately to caretakers or maintenance staff, where these exist, for action. A periodic review of environmental health facilities should also be carried out in a way that illustrates the links between the various activities. As in assessments, reviews should seek to identify causes for problems and then propose realistic solutions.

Recording forms should be developed at the level of the health-care setting, or at the district or national level for standardized monitoring reports. This will allow data from all health-care settings to be collated and compared (see the assessment checklist in Section 4).

2.10 Staff requirements and training

Infection control should be given a central place in the training and supervision of health-care workers and ancillary staff.

Many activities that are important for infection control are performed routinely by health-care workers as part of their health-care tasks. Hand hygiene is one of the most important of these activities. In smaller settings, health-care workers may also be required to perform medical and non-medical tasks, including operating and maintaining environmental health facilities.

In larger settings, other staff (such as cleaners, kitchen staff and waste technicians) are also responsible for infection control. In their training and management, they should be made aware of the importance of their role and should be able to apply the basic principles of infection control to their daily work.

Where the building design and mechanical services form part of the infection control strategy (e.g. isolation rooms, ventilation), staff training should include the importance of following correct operational procedures to ensure that protection is maintained.

2.11 Hygiene promotion

Hygiene promotion is important for staff, patients and carers. They should be given constant reminders of the importance of infection control and the routine measures required to achieve it. This applies to all health-care settings, including home care. Health promotion may be limited to providing basic information about such things as the location and correct use of toilets and handwashing points. Health-care workers have a primary role in this.

3 Guidelines for setting environmental health standards

This section contains the 11 guidelines for setting essential environmental health standards for health-care settings. These guidelines, along with their accompanying indicators, can be used to help inform or develop policies for providing health care at a national, district and local level.

3.1 Guidelines and associated information

These guidelines provide a basis for setting standards at a national level when this is required. They may be used in a similar way at district and local levels, where appropriate. The guidelines, indicators and guidance notes in this section are intended to be used, together with existing national standards and guidelines, for creating targets, policies, procedures and standards to be used in each health-care setting.

3.1.1 Guideline structure

The guidelines are given in the form of a statement that describes the situation to be aimed for and maintained. Each guideline is specified by a set of indicators that can be used as benchmark values for the following activities:

- assessing existing situations
- planning new health-care settings or improvements to existing ones
- ensuring that the construction of new health-care settings is of acceptable quality
- monitoring ongoing maintenance of facilities.

3.1.2 Indicators

The indicators are based on WHO's guidelines and have been compared with a number of other indicators from documents that also guide practice in health-care settings and other relevant settings, and are presented in the reference list. Specialist technical terms are explained in the glossary. These indicators need to be adapted in the light of national standards, local conditions and current practices. They mostly concern results — for example, the quantity of water available or the frequency of room cleaning.

3.1.3 Guidance notes

The guidance notes provide advice on applying the guidelines and indicators in practice and highlight the most important aspects that need to be considered when setting priorities for action. They are numbered according to the indicators to which they refer.

The guidelines and indicators are designed to help set targets for creating adequate conditions for the long term. Box 3.1 shows basic measures that can be taken to protect health as a temporary measure until adequate long-term conditions are provided.

> **Box 3.1 Essential temporary measures required to protect health**
>
> - Provide safe drinking-water from a protected groundwater source (spring, well or borehole), or from a treated supply, and keep it safe until it is drunk or used. Untreated water from unprotected sources can be made safer by simple means such as boiling or filtering and disinfection.
>
> - Provide water for handwashing after going to the toilet and before handling food, before and after performing health care. This may be done using simple and economical equipment, such as a pitcher of water, a basin and soap, or wood ash in some settings.
>
> - Provide basic sanitation facilities that enable patients, staff and carers to go to the toilet without contaminating the health-care setting or resources such as water supplies. This may entail measures as basic as providing simple pit latrines with reasonable privacy.
>
>   Note that the risk of transmission of soil-based helminths is increased with the use of defecation fields. The use of shoes or sandals provides protection from hookworm infections.
>
> - Provide safe health-care waste management facilities to safely contain the amount of infectious waste produced. This will require the presence of colour-coded containers in all rooms where wastes are generated.
>
> - Provide cleaning facilities that enable staff to routinely clean surfaces and fittings to ensure that the health-care environment is visibly clean and free from dust and soil. Approximately 90% of microorganisms are present within visible dirt; the purpose of cleaning is to eliminate this dirt.
>
> - Ensure that eating utensils are washed immediately after use. The sooner utensils are cleaned the easier they are to wash. Hot water and detergent, and drying on a stand are required.
>
> - Reduce the population density of disease vectors. Proper waste disposal, food hygiene, wastewater drainage, and a clean environment are key activities for controlling the presence of vectors.
>
> - Provide safe movement of air into buildings to ensure that indoor air is healthy and safe for breathing. This is particularly important if health care is being provided for people with acute respiratory diseases.
>
> - Provide information about, and implement, hygiene promotion so that staff, patients and carers are informed about essential behaviours for limiting disease transmission in health-care settings and at home.

3.2 Guidelines

> **Guideline 1 Water quality**
> Water for drinking, cooking, personal hygiene, medical activities, cleaning and laundry is safe for the purpose intended.

Indicators for Guideline 1

1. *Escherichia coli* or thermotolerant coliform bacteria are not detectable in any 100-millilitre sample of drinking-water.

   A water safety plan aimed at assessing and managing water systems, and ensuring effective operational monitoring, should be designed, developed and implemented to prevent microbial contamination in water and its ongoing safety.

2. Drinking-water meets WHO *Guidelines for drinking-water quality* (2006) or national standards concerning chemical guidelines and radiological parameters.

3. All drinking-water is treated with a residual disinfectant to ensure microbial safety up to the point of consumption or use.

4. There are no tastes, odours or colours that would discourage consumption or use of the drinking-water.

5. Water that is below drinking-water quality is used only for cleaning, laundry and sanitation and is labelled as such at every outlet.

6. Water of appropriate quality is supplied for medical activities as well as for vulnerable patients, and standards and indicators have been established.

   Pseudomonas is a recognized cause of hospital-acquired infections mainly transmitted through contact, but also through drinking-water, to immunocompromised patients (infectious dose 10^8–10^9 colony forming units/litre).

   In France, the limit value for *Legionella* concentration for patients with classical individual risk factors, such as the elderly, is < 1000 colony forming units/litre.

Guidance notes for Guideline 1

1. Microbial quality

Microbial quality is of overriding importance for infection control in health-care settings. The water should not present a risk to health from pathogens and should be protected from contamination inside the health-care setting itself. Drinking-water supplied to health-care settings should meet national standards and follow WHO guidelines for drinking-water quality (WHO, 2006). In practice, this means that the water supply should be from a protected groundwater source, such as a dug well, a borehole or a spring, or should be treated if it is from a surface water source (see Indicator 2). Rainwater may be acceptable with disinfection if the rainwater catchment surface, guttering and storage tank are correctly operated, maintained and cleaned.

Legionella spp. are common waterborne organisms, and devices such as cooling towers, hot-water systems (showers) and spas that use mains water have been associated with outbreaks of infections.

The local department of environmental health should work with the health-care setting infection control committee to monitor the microbiological quality of the water in the health-care setting, as part of a routine surveillance and control programme (WHO, 1997).

2. Chemical constituents

Chemical constituents may be present in excess of guideline levels in water supplies, and it may not be possible, in the short term, to remove them or to find an alternative source of water. In circumstances where WHO guidelines for drinking-water quality or national standards for chemical and radiological parameters cannot be met immediately, an assessment should be made of the risks caused to patients and staff, given the levels of contamination, the length of exposure (longer for staff than for patients) and the degree of susceptibility of individuals (some patients may be highly susceptible to some contaminants). It may be necessary to provide alternative sources of drinking-water for people most at risk. For example, where a water supply exceeds WHO guideline limits for nitrate or nitrite, this water should not be used for infant feeding (WHO, 2006).

3. Disinfection

Disinfection with chlorine is the most widely accepted and appropriate way of providing microbial safety in most low-cost settings. Bleaching powder, liquid bleach, chlorine tablets and other sources of chlorine may be used, depending on local availability. To ensure adequate disinfection, a contact time of at least 30 minutes should be allowed between the moment the chlorine is added to the water and the moment the water is available for consumption or use. The free chlorine residual (the free form of chlorine remaining in the water) after the contact time should be between 0.5 and 1.0 milligrams per litre (WHO, 2006) in all points of the system, including end-points. Residual chlorine can be measured with simple equipment (e.g. a colour comparator and diethyl-p-phenylenediamine tablets).

Mains supply water may need supplementary chlorination to ensure adequate disinfection and a sufficient level of residual chlorine up to the point of consumption or use. Many mains water supplies do not achieve adequate water safety at the point of delivery, due to problems at the water treatment works and contamination in the distribution system. Stored water may also need supplementary chlorination before use.

Water must not be contaminated in the health-care setting during storage, distribution and handling.

Effective disinfection requires that the water has a low turbidity. Ideally, median turbidity should be below 1 nephelometric turbidity unit (NTU) (WHO, 1997). However, 5 NTU is the minimum turbidity measurable with simple equipment (turbidity tube), so this level may be used in low-cost settings in practice. If turbidity exceeds 5 NTU then the water should be treated to remove suspended matter before disinfection, by sedimentation (with or without coagulation and flocculation) and/or filtration.

Filtration with ceramic (e.g. candle filters), chlorination and other technologies that can be used on a small scale may be appropriate for treating water in health-care settings that are not connected to piped supplies, as well as those that are connected to piped supplies whose quality is not consistently satisfactory (WHO, 2002a).

4. Drinking-water quality

Drinking-water should be acceptable to patients and staff, or they may not drink enough, or may drink water from other, unprotected sources, which could be harmful to their health.

Particular care is needed to ensure that safe drinking-water is supplied to immunocompromised patients, because of their high susceptibility to infection. Provision of boiled water may be desirable.

5. Water for cleaning

Water used for laundry and for cleaning floors and other surfaces need not be of drinking-water quality, as long as it is used with a disinfectant or a detergent.

6. Water for medical purposes

Water used for some medical activities may need to be of higher quality. For example, water used for haemodialysis should meet strict criteria concerning microbial contamination and chemical contaminants, including chlorine and aluminium, which are commonly used in drinking-water treatment.

> **Guideline 2 Water quantity**
> Sufficient water is available at all times for drinking, food preparation, personal hygiene, medical activities, cleaning and laundry.

Indicators for Guideline 2

1. Minimum water quantity required[5]

    Table 3.1, below, lists the minimum quantity of water that is required for different situations in the health-care setting.

Table 3.1 Minimum water quantities required in the health-care setting

Outpatients	5 litres/consultation
Inpatients	40–60 litres/patient/day
Operating theatre or maternity unit	100 litres/intervention
Dry or supplementary feeding centre	0.5–5 litres/consultation (depending on waiting time)

---

[5] According to situations (e.g. for use of a flush toilet, the water requirement can be much higher).

Wet supplementary feeding centre	15 litres/consultation
Inpatient therapeutic feeding centre	30 litres/patient/day
Cholera treatment centre	60 litres/patient/day
Severe acute respiratory diseases isolation centre	100 litres/patient/day
Viral haemorrhagic fever isolation centre	300–400 litres/patient/day

Guidance notes for Guideline 2

1. Use of minimum water quantities

These guideline volumes include water used for all purposes: hand hygiene, cleaning, laundry, drinking and cooking. The figures should be used for planning and designing water supply systems. The actual quantities of water required will depend on a number of factors, such as climate, availability and type of water use facilities (including type of toilets), level of care and local water use practices.

Although figures are provided for the isolation and treatment of patients with cholera, severe acute respiratory syndrome and viral haemorrhagic fever, these account for relatively few hospitalizations.

> **Guideline 3   Water facilities and access to water**
> Sufficient water-collection points and water-use facilities are available in the health-care setting to allow convenient access to, and use of, water for medical activities, drinking, personal hygiene, food preparation, laundry and cleaning.

Indicators for Guideline 3

1. A reliable drinking-water point is accessible for staff, patients and carers at all times.

2. A reliable water point, with soap or a suitable alternative, is available at all critical points within the health-care setting (operating theatres, wards, consulting rooms, dressing stations, etc.) and in service areas (sterilization, laboratory, kitchen, laundry, showers, toilets, waste zone and mortuary).

3. At least two handwashing basins should be provided in wards with more than 20 beds.

4. At least one shower is available for 40 users in inpatient settings (users include patients, staff and carers staying in the health-care setting).

5. Laundry facilities, with soap or detergent, hot water and a disinfectant (such as chlorine solution), are available for inpatient settings.

Guidance notes for Guideline 3

1. Drinking-water points

Drinking-water should be provided separately from water provided for handwashing and other purposes, even if it is from the same supply. Drinking-water may be provided from a piped water system or via a covered container with a tap where there is no piped supply. Drinking-water points should be clearly marked.

2. Handwashing

Basic hygiene measures by staff, patients and carers, handwashing in particular, should not be compromised by lack of water.

Waterless, alcohol-based handrubs may be used for rapid, repeated decontamination of clean hands. Handrub dispensers can be installed at convenient points, and can also be carried by staff as they move between patients. However, handrubs may not be affordable, and they do not replace soap and water for cleaning soiled hands.

3. Handwashing facilities

Water points should be sufficiently close to users to encourage them to use water as often as required. Alternatively, a handwashing basin, soap and a jug of clean water may be placed on a trolley used for ward rounds, to encourage handwashing as often as needed between patient contacts.

4. Showering facilities

Although less important than handwashing in terms of reducing disease transmission, showering (or other means of washing the body) may be important for the recovery of certain patients, and may be required by staff and carers in contact with infectious patients.

If piped hot water is available, measures should be taken to avoid the proliferation of bacteria in the water system. For this reason, piped water and water from showers should ideally be maintained below 20°C or above 50°C.[6]

Separate showers may be needed for staff and patients, and for both sexes, to ensure that all groups have adequate privacy and safety.

5. Laundry facilities

See Guideline 7 for more details.

---

[6] Specific cleaning and disinfection procedures against *Pseudomonas* and possibly *Legionella* have to be foreseen.

> **Guideline 4   Excreta disposal**
> Adequate, accessible and appropriate toilets are provided for patients, staff and carers.

Indicators for Guideline 4

1. There are sufficient toilets available: one per 20 users for inpatient settings; at least four toilets per outpatient setting (one for staff, and for patients: one for females, one for males and one for children).

2. Toilets are appropriate for local technical and financial conditions.

3. Toilets are designed to respond to local cultural and social conditions and all age and user groups.

4. Toilets are safe to use.

5. Toilets have convenient handwashing facilities close by.

6. Toilets are easily accessible (that is, no more than 30 metres from all users).

7. There is a cleaning and maintenance routine in operation that ensures that clean and functioning toilets are available at all times.

Guidance notes for Guideline 4

1.   Ratio of people per toilet

The recommended ratio of one toilet per 20 people is common and widespread, and should be used as a planning guideline. Actual numbers required for inpatient settings will depend on a number of factors, including the average proportion of patients using bedpans instead of toilets. Users include patients, staff and carers.

In outpatient settings, a suitable arrangement is often as follows: one toilet for staff (two if separate toilets are required for male and female staff), one toilet for male patients, one toilet for female patients, and one child's toilet. In larger outpatient settings, more toilets are required. The number required depends on a number of local factors, including the average time patients wait before consultations.

2.   Local technical and financial conditions

If there is sufficient and reliable piped water available and there is a connection to a sewer system or a functioning septic tank and drainage system, flush toilets may be appropriate, depending on materials used for anal cleansing. In other situations, latrines (dry or pour-flush types) are appropriate. Care must be taken, when siting latrines, to avoid contaminating groundwater and risk of flooding.

3.   Social and cultural considerations

In most cases, separate toilets are required for men and women, and separate toilets should be provided for staff and patients. They should be clearly signposted to help users find them.

Patient toilets should be equipped to make them easy to use by people with physical handicaps, heavily pregnant women, elderly people and people who are sick (see e.g. Jones and Reed 2005 for detailed design features).

Special children's toilets should be provided where many children use the health-care setting. Children's toilets are particularly useful where latrines are used and where the size of the drop hole and the conditions inside a normal latrine are off-putting for children or inconvenient for carers.

Toilets should be designed and equipped to respond to cultural identities (e.g. anal cleansing with water).

4. Hygiene and safety concerns

Toilets should be designed, built and maintained so that they are hygienic and acceptable to use and do not become centres for disease transmission. This includes measures to control fly and mosquito breeding, and a regularly monitored cleaning schedule.

In order to minimize the risk of violence, including sexual violence, toilets should be carefully located, should be lockable by the user (to protect people while using them), and they and their access routes should be lit at night.

5. Handwashing points

Water points, with soap and adequate drainage, should be provided at the exit of all toilets, and their use should be actively encouraged.

6. Accessibility

Time and effort required to reach the toilets need to be taken into account. In multi-storey buildings, there should be toilets available on all floors, and routes used to reach toilets should be smooth and flat, for easy access for people in wheelchairs.

7. Cleaning and maintenance

Toilets should be cleaned whenever they are dirty, and at least twice per day, with a disinfectant used on all exposed surfaces and a brush to remove visible soiling. Strong disinfectants should not be used in large quantities, as this is unnecessary, expensive, potentially dangerous, and may affect the biodegradation process. If no disinfectant is available, plain cold water should be used.

In specific contexts (e.g. isolation for cholera patients), a 2% active chlorine solution is used to disinfect faeces or vomit. Usually the chlorine solution is already contained in the container that will receive the faeces or vomit from the patients in bed.

Guideline 5   Wastewater disposal
Wastewater is disposed of rapidly and safely.

Indicators for Guideline 5

1. Wastewater is removed rapidly and cleanly from the point where it is produced.

2. Wastewater drainage from health-care settings is built and managed to avoid contamination of the health-care setting or the broader environment.

3. Rainwater and surface run-off is safely disposed of and does not carry contamination from the health-care setting to the outside surrounding environment.

Guidance notes for Guideline 5

1.   Wastewater drainage systems

Wastewater is produced from washbasins, showers, sinks, etc. (grey water) and from flushing toilets (black water). It should be removed in standard waste drainage systems to off-site sewer or on-site disposal systems. All open wastewater drainage systems should be covered, to avoid the risks of disease vector breeding and contamination from direct exposure.

Small quantities of infectious liquid wastes (e.g. blood or body fluids) may be poured into sinks or toilets. Most pathogens are inactivated by a combination of time, dilution and the presence of disinfectants in the wastewater. Toxic wastes (e.g. reagents from a laboratory) should be treated as health-care waste (see Guideline 6). They should not be poured into sinks or toilets that drain into the wastewater system.

2.   Prevention of environmental contamination

The most appropriate wastewater disposal option is connecting the health-care setting to a properly built and functioning sewer system, which is, in turn, connected to an adequate treatment plant.

If the sewer does not lead to a treatment facility, an on-site retention system with treatment will be necessary before wastewater is discharged.

In other situations, on-site disposal is needed. For grey water, soakaway pits or infiltration trenches should be used. These should be equipped with grease traps, which should be checked weekly and cleaned, if needed, to ensure the systems operate correctly. Pits or trenches should not overflow into the health-care setting grounds or surroundings and create insect or rodent breeding sites. Black water should be disposed of in a septic tank, with the effluent discharged into a soakaway pit or infiltration trench. Grey and black water may be treated in the same septic tank and soakaway system, although this requires a larger septic tank than one used for black water alone. All systems that infiltrate wastewater into the ground should be sited so as to avoid contaminating groundwater. There should be at least 1.5 metres between the bottom of the infiltration system and the groundwater table (more in coarse sands, gravels and fissured formations), and the system should be at least 30 metres from any groundwater source.

If the health-care setting has a septic tank, the sludge from the tank should not be used for agricultural purposes, but should be buried following safe procedures.

3. Rainwater and surface run-off

Rainwater and surface run-off may be drained and disposed of separately if the system in place for wastewater cannot cope with additional water from sudden heavy rains or rainwater and surface run-off. In that case, it must be managed in a way that does not carry contamination from the health-care setting to the outside surrounding. Correct, separate drainage of rainwater is particularly important for settings such as cholera treatment centres where there is a high prevalence of enteric pathogens that might be washed out of the isolation area into the local environment.

> **Guideline 6 Health-care waste disposal**
> Health-care waste is segregated, collected, transported, treated and disposed of safely.

Indicators for Guideline 6

1. Health-care waste is segregated at the point of generation according to its type, using four major categories: sharps, non-sharps infectious waste, non-sharps non-infectious waste and hazardous waste.

2. Colour-coded waste containers or containers bearing clearly understood signs and symbols are provided at convenient locations. They are collected from all health-care services and stored safely before treatment and/or disposal.

3. Each category of waste is treated and disposed of according to the safest feasible method available.

4. A specific waste-disposal zone exists, where wastes can be stored and disposed of safely and effectively.

Guidance notes for Guideline 6

1. Segregation

The four major categories of health-care waste recommended for organizing segregation and separate storage, collection and disposal are:

- sharps (needles, scalpels, etc.), which may be infectious or not
- non-sharps infectious waste (anatomical waste, pathological waste, dressings, used syringes, used single-use gloves)
- non-sharps non-infectious waste (paper, packaging, etc.)
- hazardous waste (expired drugs, laboratory reagents, radioactive waste, insecticides, etc.).

2. Storage and collection

Sharps should be placed immediately in yellow puncture-proof and covered safe sharps containers, which are regularly collected for disposal.

Non-sharps infectious yellow or red waste bags or containers (15–40-litre capacity, with lids) should be collected, emptied, cleaned, disinfected and replaced after each intervention (e.g. in an operating or maternity unit) or twice daily.

Non-sharps non-infectious black waste containers (20–60 litre capacity) should be collected, emptied, cleaned and replaced daily; alternatively, plastic bags may be used inside the containers.

For the above categories of waste, it is recommended that waste containers are a maximum of 5 metres from the point of waste generation, in two sets for each location, for a minimum of three types of waste. At least one set of waste containers should be provided per 20 beds in a ward.

Hazardous waste should be collected and stored in appropriate and labelled containers placed in secure location. Radioactive waste should be stored in containers that prevent dispersion, behind lead shielding.

3. Treatment and disposal

Sharps should be disposed of in a sharps pit (buried drums in small health centres or emergency structures; concrete-lined pits in other settings). Off-site treatment in a decentralised facility in charge of collection, treatment and disposal is not advisable for safety reasons but may be necessary in an urban area where on-site treatment is not feasible because of lack of space.

Non-sharps infectious waste should be buried in a pit fitted with a sealed cover and ventilation pipe for on-site treatment in small health-care settings or, should be high-temperature incinerated or steam sterilized on-site or off-site. Special arrangements may be needed for disposing of placentas, according to local custom.

The preferred option for specific infectious waste (such as blood samples, plastic syringes and laboratory tests) is steam sterilization before disposal, if available. This avoids environmental pollution from incineration. One autoclave should be dedicated for waste sterilization, different from the autoclave used for sterilizing medical devices within the laboratory (see e.g. Diaz and Savage (2003) for details on a range of processes for treating infectious wastes).

Non-sharps non-infectious waste should be buried in a pit, a landfill site or preferably recycled in non-food and non-medical items. If space is limited, non-sharps non-infectious waste should be incinerated. Ashes and residues should be buried in a pit.

There are several kinds of hazardous waste and each requires specific treatment and disposal methods, which include encapsulation, sterilization, burial, incineration and long-term storage. Some wastes, such as pharmaceutical wastes, cannot be disposed of in low-cost settings and should be sent to a large centre for destruction or returned to the supplier. In all cases, national legislation should be followed.

4. Waste-disposal zone

The waste-disposal zone should be fenced off; it should have a water point with soap or detergent and disinfectant for handwashing or to clean and disinfect containers, with facilities for wastewater disposal into a soakaway system or sewer. The waste-disposal zone should also be located at least 30 metres from groundwater sources. Where an incinerator is used, it should be located to allow effective operation with minimal local air pollution in the health centre, nearby housing and crops, and it should be large enough for extension if new pits or other facilities have to be built.

Guideline 7	Cleaning and laundry

Laundry and surfaces in the health-care environment are kept clean.

Indicators for Guideline 7

1. Routine programmed cleaning of surfaces and fittings is carried out to ensure that the health-care environment is visibly clean, and free from dust and soil. All horizontal surfaces are cleaned at least daily and whenever they are soiled.

2. The intensity of cleanliness maintained is appropriate to the likelihood of contamination and the degree of asepsis required.

3. Any areas contaminated with blood or body fluids are cleaned and disinfected immediately.

4. Soiled linen is placed in appropriate bags at the point of generation and pre-disinfected, washed in water, rinsed and dried in a covered place.

5. Clean and soiled linen are transported and stored separately, in different (marked) bags.

6. Beds, mattresses and pillows are cleaned between patients and whenever soiled with body fluids.

Guidance notes for Guideline 7

1. Routine cleaning

Ninety per cent of microorganisms are present within visible dirt, which should be eliminated by routine cleaning. Neither ordinary soap nor detergents have antimicrobial activity, and the cleaning process depends essentially on mechanical action. Wet mopping with hot water and detergent, if available, is recommended, rather than sweeping (WHO, 2002b). If hot water is not available, a 0.2 % chlorine solution, or other suitable disinfectant in cold water should be used. However, detergent is sufficient for normal, domestic cleaning of floors and other surfaces that are not in contact with hands and medical instruments.

2. Intensity of cleaning routine

Floors and other washed surfaces should be made of a suitable, non-porous material that is resistant to repeated cleaning with hot water and detergents or disinfectants. This may be achieved by classifying areas of the health-care setting into three areas, each with a specific cleaning routine (WHO, 2002b):

- *Sweeping*: offices and other non-patient areas; normal daily domestic cleaning.

- *Wet mopping daily*: waiting areas, consulting rooms, non-infectious disease wards, pharmacy.

- *Cleaning with a detergent or disinfectant solution, with separate cleaning equipment for each room daily, whenever soiled and after each intervention (in the case of operating suites and delivery rooms)*: infectious disease or isolation wards, protective isolation wards for highly susceptible patients and protected areas, such as operating suites, delivery rooms, intensive care units, premature baby units, casualty departments, haemodialysis units, laboratory, laundry, kitchen, sterilization services.

In cholera treatment settings, a 0.2 % chlorine solution or other disinfectant should be used for cleaning floors, walls and beds daily and whenever soiled. Soiled clothing and bedding should be disinfected in 0.2 % chlorine solution for 10 minutes and then rinsed, before being washed and dried as usual.

3. Blood or body fluids

Chlorine solution (1%) is adequate for cleaning and disinfecting blood or body fluid spills. Large spills should first be removed with absorbent material (which should then be properly disposed of; see Guideline 6), before disinfecting and cleaning.

4. Cleaning soiled linen

Soiled linen should not be sorted in patient-care areas, and should be handled with minimum agitation to avoid releasing pathogens. Soiled linen should be cleaned and autoclaved before being supplied to operating rooms or theatres. Woollen blankets should be washed in warm water (WHO, 2004b).

5. Transporting soiled linen

Securely closed impermeable bags should be used for transporting linen heavily soiled with body substances or other fluids (WHO, 2004b).

6. Beds and bedding

Beds should be wiped with a disinfectant solution (e.g. 0.2% chlorine solution) following each hospitalization.

Mattresses should have waterproof protective covers for easy cleaning. Mattresses and pillows should be treated, as required, to control lice, bedbugs and other nuisances or disease vectors.

If woven mats are used instead of, or on top of, mattresses, they should be destroyed (burned) and replaced between patients.

If insecticide-treated nets are used on beds, they should be washed and reimpregnated every 6 months if used only for patients with non-infectious diseases. If used for patients with infectious diseases (cholera, haemorrhagic fevers, etc.), they should be washed and reimpregnated between patients and whenever soiled. Non insecticide-treated net should be impregnated.

> **Guideline 8   Food storage and preparation**
>
> Food for patients, staff and carers is stored and prepared in a way that minimizes the risk of disease transmission.
>
> The information in these indicators and guidance notes is drawn from WHO (2001) and WHO (2004c).

Indicators for Guideline 8

1. Food handling and preparation is done with utmost cleanliness.

2. Contact between raw foodstuffs and cooked food is avoided.

3. Food is cooked thoroughly.

4. Food is kept at safe temperatures.

5. Safe water and raw ingredients are used.

6. Powdered infant formula is prepared appropriately.

Guidance notes for Guideline 8

1. Food handling and preparation

Food handlers should be trained in basic food safety.

Food handlers should wash their hands after using the toilet and whenever they start work, change tasks, or return after an interruption. Soap and water should be available at all times during food preparation and handling, to ensure that handwashing can be done conveniently (see Guidance note 3).

Kitchen staff and carers with colds, influenza, diarrhoea, vomiting and throat and skin infections, or those who have suffered from diarrhoea and vomiting within the past 48 hours, should not handle food unless it is packaged. All infections should be reported and sick staff should not be penalised.

Food-preparation premises should be kept meticulously clean. Surfaces used for food preparation should be washed with detergent and safe water and then rinsed, or wiped with a clean cloth that is frequently washed. Scraps of food should be disposed of rapidly, as they are potential reservoirs for bacteria and can attract insects and rodents. Refuse should be kept in covered bins and disposed of quickly and safely (see Guideline 6).

Eating utensils should be washed immediately after each use with hot water and detergent, and air-dried. The sooner utensils are cleaned the easier they are to wash. Drying cloths should not be used, as they can spread contamination.

In many inpatient settings, carers may bring food to patients, or may prepare food at the health-care setting. In these cases, staff should seek to ensure that food is prepared hygienically and that cooked food is consumed immediately. Cooking facilities may need to be provided.

2. **Separation of food and equipment**

Separate equipment and utensils, such as knives and cutting boards, should be used for handling raw foods or they should be washed and sanitized in between uses.

Food should be stored in containers to avoid contact between raw and prepared foods.

Raw meat, poultry and seafood should be separated from other foods.

3. **Cooking and serving**

All parts of foods cooked must reach 70°C to kill dangerous microorganisms. To ensure this happens, soups and stews should be brought to the boil and meat should be heated until juices are clear, not pink.

Cooked food must be reheated thoroughly to steaming hot all the way through.

Cooked food to be served should be kept hot (more than 60°C) before serving.

4. **Storage**

Cooked or perishable food should not be left at room temperature for more than two hours, and should be prepared or supplied fresh each day. All food should be kept covered to protect it from flies and dust.

Non-perishable foods should be stored safely in a closed, dry, well-ventilated store and protected from rodents and insects. They should not be stored in the same room as pesticides, disinfectants or any other toxic chemicals. Containers that have previously held toxic chemicals should not be used for storing foodstuffs.

Bought food should not be used beyond its expiry date.

Food should be protected from insects, rodents and other animals, which frequently carry pathogenic organisms and are a potential source of contamination of food (see Guideline 10).

5. **Washing and use of water**

Only safe water should be used for food preparation, handwashing and cleaning. For specification of safe water, see Guideline 1.

Fruit and vegetables should be washed with safe water. If there is any doubt about the cleanliness of raw fruit and vegetables, they should be peeled.

6. Powdered infant formula

Powdered infant formula should be prepared with water that is not cooler that 70°C (in order to kill *Enterobacter sakazakii*), stored and handled in accordance with *How to prepare powdered infant formula in care settings* (WHO and FAO, 2007).[7]

> **Guideline 9   Building design, construction and management**
> Buildings are designed, constructed and managed to provide a healthy and comfortable environment for patients, staff and carers.

Indicators for Guideline 9

1. The air temperature, humidity and airflow in the health-care setting provide a comfortable environment for patients, staff and carers.

2. Airflow minimizes the risk of transmission of airborne pathogens from infected patients and minimizes risks to susceptible staff, patients and carers.

3. Sufficient lighting is provided during all working hours to allow safe movement of staff, patients and carers, and normal undertaking of medical activities.

4. Buildings are designed and activities are organized so as to minimize the spread of contamination by the movement of patients, staff and carers, equipment, supplies and contaminated items, including health-care waste, and to facilitate hygiene.

5. Health-care settings are built, furnished and equipped with materials that minimize infectious disease transmission and facilitate cleaning.

6. Sufficient space is provided for people in wheelchairs, as well as to minimize infectious disease transmission.

Guidance notes for Guideline 9

1. Ventilation

Guideline 9 should be followed by locating and constructing buildings that use designs and materials that produce the best indoor conditions, taking into account the local climate and prevailing winds.

---

[7] WHO recommends that infants are exclusively breastfed for the first six months of life to achieve optimal growth, development and health. There are instances where breast milk is not available; where the mother is unable to breastfeed; where she has made an informed decision not to breastfeed; or — for example — where the mother is taking medication that is contraindicated for breastfeeding, or the mother is HIV-positive. Similarly, some very low-birth-weight babies may not be able to breastfeed directly, and in some cases, expressed breast milk may not be available at all or available in insufficient quantities. Infants who are not breastfed require a suitable breast-milk substitute, for example, infant formula.

The effective use of blinds, opening and closing of doors and windows, planting of suitable vegetation around the building and other operational measures can help optimize indoor conditions.

In addition to basic construction and operation measures, heating, ventilation and air-conditioning, or filters may be required for specific areas or activities of the health-care setting. If heating, ventilation and air-conditioning, or filters are used, they should be maintained regularly to ensure their continued effectiveness. Filters should be inspected regularly and cleaned or changed as required, because biofilms may build up and become breeding places for microorganisms, resulting in, for example, health-care acquired *Legionella* transmission. Ceiling fans and small portable ventilators are not recommended as they dispense dust around the room (especially over the sterile field and equipment in an operating theatre).

2. Air extraction to minimize pathogens

Minimizing the risk of transmission of airborne pathogens from infected patients may require isolation in a negative-air-pressure room, where air is drawn into the room and extracted by a fan, thus avoiding contaminated air circulating to other parts of the health-care setting. Care should be taken when siting the air extractor for an isolation room to reduce the risk of transmission to people outside the building and to minimize the risk of the contaminated air being drawn into another area of the building by other parts of the ventilation system.

Operating theatres and rooms for isolating particularly vulnerable patients (e.g. severely immunocompromised patients) may require positive air pressure conditions, where clean air is drawn into the room, thus avoiding contaminated air entering from other parts of the health-care setting.

In both negative and positive pressure facilities, operational procedures should be drawn up (e.g. ensuring doors are closed and that ventilation is operational) and staff should be properly trained to ensure correct operation of the room. In negative-pressure facilities, the risk of transmission to nursing staff may be significant and additional protective measures, such as masks, should be used routinely.

All occupied areas of the health-care facility should be adequately ventilated to meet comfort requirements. Where infected and susceptible people share the same air space and there is a risk of airborne transmission of infection, ventilation rates should be maximized to dilute and remove any infectious particles. Guidelines for the control of tuberculosis transmission in high-risk locations recommend that mechanically ventilated spaces have an air change rate of 6–12 air changes per hour (Jensen et al. 2005). While this is not feasible in many low-cost settings, high ventilation rates are possible with natural ventilation (Escombe et al. 2007), and where the climate allows, large opening windows, skylights and other vents can be used to optimize natural ventilation.

Where possible, air should flow into rooms from the top and out of the room from the bottom (near the floor, which is generally the most likely contaminated part of the room), and natural ventilation should be optimized wherever feasible.

3. Lighting

Natural light may be sufficient in outpatient settings that operate only during the day. However, some form of lighting should be available for night-time emergencies.

In isolated inpatient settings (such as rural hospitals) and in temporary structures (such as cholera treatment centres), generators or solar panels and batteries are likely to be required and provision for these should be made. As a minimum, a safe type of kerosene or gas lantern and powerful hand torches should be available.

4. Movement between areas

Given the size and complexity of the health-care setting and the resources available, activities should be organized in zones, with the flow of people, equipment and materials managed so as to minimize movements from "dirty" to "clean" zones.

Services should be located in relation to each other so as to facilitate hygienic management. For instance, the sterilization service should be close to the operating theatre.

5. Cleaning

All surfaces should be easy to clean by wet mopping and should be able to withstand repeated exposure to hot water, detergents and disinfectants.

Walls, floors and ceiling surfaces should be smooth and made of non-porous materials that are easy to clean and that do not provide a suitable environment for pathogen survival or development. The same is true for furniture and equipment used for patient care.

6. Building design

The building of new health-care settings or the improvement of existing ones should be in line with national building codes and standard health-care setting building designs. For example, beds for patients should be separated by a minimum of one metre and should be easily accessible by people with physical handicaps or elderly people.

Guideline 10   Control of vector-borne disease
Patients, staff and carers are protected from disease vectors.

Indicators for Guideline 10

1. The number of vectors in the health-care setting is minimized.

2. Patients, staff and carers are protected from potential disease-transmitting vectors.

3. Spread of vector-borne diseases is minimized by preventing contact with infected substances or materials.

Guidance notes for Guideline 10

1. Minimizing disease vectors

Appropriate and effective methods for excluding or reducing vector numbers depend on the type of vector; the location and number or size of breeding sites; vector habits, including places and times of resting, feeding and biting; and resistance of specific vector populations to control chemicals.

Basic environmental control methods, such as proper drainage, waste disposal and food hygiene, should be the basis of any strategy (see *Legionella and the prevention of legionellosis*, WHO 2007).

Mosquitoes and flies can effectively be excluded from buildings by covering opening windows with fly screens and fitting self-closing doors to the outside.

Any use of chemical controls requires specialist advice, such as for residual insecticide spraying, in and around the health-care setting. Advice should be available from within the ministry of health.

2. **Protect patients and staff from vector-borne diseases**

Once inside the health-care setting, patients, staff and carers may be protected from certain vectors through the use of barriers (e.g. insecticide bednets against mosquitoes or covered food storage to prevent contamination by rats and flies) or repellents.

Patients with vector-borne diseases, such as malaria, Lassa fever and typhus, should be treated or protected to ensure that the related vectors do not transmit the disease from them to other people in the health-care setting. This may require removal of the vectors (e.g. insecticide dusting to remove lice from typhus patients) or the use of a barrier (e.g. insecticide bednets to isolate yellow fever patients from mosquitoes).

3. **Prevent spread of vectors**

Infectious substances such as excreta and soiled dressings should be disposed of immediately and completely to prevent flies and other mechanical vectors from carrying pathogens to food, eyes, wounds, etc., or distributing them to the environment.

> **Guideline 11   Information and hygiene promotion**
> Correct use of water, sanitation and waste facilities is encouraged by hygiene promotion and by management of staff, patients and carers.

Indicators for Guideline 11

1. Staff are trained and managed in a way that encourages consistent compliance with infection control procedures.

2. Patients and carers are informed about essential behaviours necessary for limiting disease transmission in the health-care setting and in the home.

3. Facilities and resources enable staff, patients and carers to practise behaviours that control disease transmission in an easy and timely way.

Guidance notes for Guideline 11

1. **Training in infection control**

Infection control should be a core part of initial training, and refresher trainings should be carried out regularly to sustain knowledge and awareness of staff.

Infection control should be highlighted as an institutional priority, and a climate that encourages patient and staff safety should be developed.

As part of an infection control strategy, all staff, once sufficiently trained and equipped, should be sanctioned for non-compliance with reasonable procedures. They should be updated on any changes. In particular, senior staff should provide role models by complying consistently with procedures.

All staff at risk should be vaccinated against hepatitis B (WHO, 2002b).

2. Behaviours for limiting disease transmission

Information about behaviours for limiting disease transmission should be provided verbally by staff, who should have the time to explain clearly to patients and carers.

Posters and other visual information should be used to promote disease control among patients and carers. Visual information should be relevant to risk practices, it should be understood by the target audience and it should provide practical and realistic advice and information.

Patients' and carers' contact with the health-care setting should be used as a means to promote hygiene in the community. Both during normal periods and during epidemics, health-care settings should be actively involved in preventive health care through hygiene promotion.

3. Adequate facilities

Staff, patients and carers should not be expected to adopt behaviours that are inconvenient, uncomfortable or impractical. For example, staff are unlikely to comply fully with handwashing procedures if there are no handwashing facilities close to where they care for patients (WHO, advanced draft). Refer to Guidelines 1 to 10.

4 Assessment checklist

The following checklist provides a set of assessment questions for each of the guidelines presented in Section 3, to measure the extent to which the guidelines are followed and identify areas for action. The qualitative and quantitative indicators under the relevant guideline can be used as references to help answer the questions. Questions may be answered with a "yes", a "no" or a "not applicable". A "no" answer to any question should alert the assessor that remedial action is required, either in the design and construction of facilities or their operation and maintenance. Guidance on action to take can be found in the guidance notes under each guideline in Section 3.

1   Water quality

Water for drinking, cooking, personal hygiene, medical activities, cleaning and laundry is safe for the purpose intended

	Design and construction	Operation and maintenance
1	• Is water from a safe source (free from faecal contamination)? • Is water protected from contamination in the HCS?	• Is the safety of the water source monitored regularly? • Is the quality of the water supplied to the HCS monitored regularly? • Are water storage, distribution and use facilities in the HCS adequately maintained to avoid contaminating the water?
2	• If necessary, can water be treated at the HCS?	• If water is treated at the HCS, is the treatment process operated effectively? • Are there sufficient supplies and adequately trained staff to carry out treatment? • Is the quality of the treated water monitored regularly? • Are treatment processes monitored regularly?
3	• Does the water supply meet WHO guidelines or national standards regarding chemical or radiological parameters?	• If necessary, are measures in place to avoid overexposure of susceptible patients to chemical contaminants?
4	• Is water acceptable (smell, taste, appearance)?	• If the water is not acceptable is there a safe alternative supply of drinking-water?
5	• Is the water supply designed and built so that low-quality water used for cleaning, laundry, etc. cannot enter the drinking-water supply and is identified as non-potable at all outlets?	• Are procedures in place for keeping both water supplies independent and well identified, and are procedures followed consistently?

HCS, health-care setting; WHO, World Health Organization

2 Water quantity

Sufficient water is available at all times for drinking, food preparation, personal hygiene, medical activities, cleaning and laundry

	Design and construction	Operation and maintenance
1	• Does the water supply have the capacity required? • Is there a suitable alternative supply in case of need?	• Is sufficient water available at all times for all needs? • Is the water supply operated and maintained to prevent wastage?

3 Water facilities and access to water

Sufficient water-collection points and water-use facilities are available in the health centre to allow convenient access to, and use of, water for drinking, food preparation, personal hygiene, medical activities, laundry and cleaning

	Design and construction	Operation and maintenance
1	• Are there sufficient, clearly identified drinking-water points?	• Are drinking-water points properly used and adequately maintained?
2	• Are there sufficient water points in the right place for all needs?	• Is water accessible where needed at all times?
3	• Are handwashing points available in all areas where health-care is carried out?	• Is there always soap or a suitable alternative at handwashing points?
4	• In inpatient HCSs, are there sufficient showers?	• Are showers properly used and adequately maintained?
5	• In inpatient HCSs, are there sufficient laundry facilities?	• Are laundry facilities properly used and adequately maintained?

HCS, health-care setting

4   Excreta disposal

Adequate, accessible and appropriate toilets are provided for patients, staff and carers

	Design and construction	Operation and maintenance
1	• Are there sufficient toilets in the health-care setting?	• Are there sufficient toilets actually in use?
2	• Are the toilets technically adapted to local maintenance systems? • Are the toilets affordable in the short term and long term?	• Are the toilets maintained and repaired in a timely and effective way?
3	• Are the toilets designed to suit local culture and social conditions? • Do the toilets provide privacy and security?	• Do patients, staff and carers find the toilets appropriate? • Are the toilets used according to their design?
4	• Are the toilets hygienic to use and easy to clean?	• Are the toilets clean and without smell?
5	• Are there handwashing facilities close by the toilets?	• Is there water and soap available all the time?
6	• Are the toilets easily accessible for all users?	• Are access routes to toilets kept in good condition and well lit?
7	• Is there a cleaning and maintenance plan?	• Is there an effective cleaning and maintenance routine in operation?

5   Wastewater disposal

Wastewater is disposed of rapidly and safely

	Design and construction	Operation and maintenance
1	• Does the wastewater drainage system have sufficient capacity? • Does the system have the correct design (drainage slopes, etc.)?	• Is the system operated and cleaned so as to maintain its capacity?
2	• Is the system designed and built so as to protect the broader environment?	• Are protective features (e.g. grease traps) properly maintained?
3	• Does the rainwater and surface run-off drainage system avoid carrying contamination outside the health-care setting?	• Are cleaning and wastewater disposal activities prevented from ending up in the open environment and contaminating rainwater and run-off?

6   Health-care waste disposal

Health-care waste is segregated, collected, transported, treated and disposed of safely

	Design and construction	Operation and maintenance
1	• Are there facilities in place for segregating health-care waste at the point of generation?	• Are the segregation facilities used effectively?
2	• Are there sufficient waste containers of the right sort and design in the right places?	• Are waste containers emptied, cleaned and replaced (or disposed of) frequently enough?
3	• Are there appropriate treatment and disposal facilities in place for the quantity and nature of health-care waste produced?	• Are the treatment and disposal facilities correctly operated and maintained? • Are waste-related injuries along the waste-management chain correctly reported and acted on?
4	• Is there a specific waste-disposal zone with the necessary features?	• Is the waste-disposal zone operated so as to prevent contamination?

7 Cleaning and laundry

Laundry and surfaces in the health-care environment are kept clean

	Design and construction	Operation and maintenance
1	• Are washed surfaces made of non-porous and resistant material?	• Are surfaces and fittings cleaned routinely? Are they visibly clean?
2	• Are the cleaning requirements of different zones of the HCS defined?	• Are different zones of the HCS cleaned according to their specific requirements?
3	• Are the cleaning requirements for blood and body fluids well defined?	• Are contaminated spills cleaned and disinfected immediately?
4	• Are there sufficient laundry facilities at the HCS?	• Is soiled linen placed immediately in bags and then correctly washed and dried?
5	• Are there sufficient bags and storage facilities for clean and soiled linen?	• Is clean and soiled linen transported and stored separately?
6	• Do mattresses have waterproof covers?	• Are mattresses and pillows cleaned between patients and whenever soiled? • If mats are used, are they destroyed and replaced between patients?
7	• Is appropriate equipment available for cleaning, disinfection and sterilization of medical equipment?	• Is medical equipment appropriately cleaned and then disinfected or sterilized between uses?

HCS, health-care setting

8 Food storage and preparation

Food for patients, staff and carers is stored and prepared so as to minimize the risk of disease transmission

	Design and construction	Operation and maintenance
1	• Are there handwashing points in the food preparation area and at the toilets that food handlers use?	• Do food handlers wash their hands when necessary?
2	• Are food storage and preparation areas designed and built so as to be easy to keep clean?	• Are food preparation areas kept clean and protected from rodents and insects?
3	• Are there facilities and equipment provided for preventing contact between cooked and raw foodstuffs?	• Is contact between raw foodstuffs and cooked food prevented?
4	• Are cooking facilities adequate for heating food sufficiently?	• Is food cooked thoroughly?
5	• If cooked food or raw ingredients are stored, is there a fridge at the HCS for this?	• Is food kept at safe temperatures?
6	• If dry foods are stored at the HCS, is the store appropriate?	• Are dry food stores kept clean and protected from rodents and insects?
7	• Do facilities exist to allow the safe preparation, storage and handling of powdered infant formula?	• Is powdered infant formula prepared with hot water that is not cooler than 70°C, stored and handled according to the WHO and FAO (2007) guidelines?

HCS, health-care setting

9 Building design, construction and management

Buildings are designed, constructed and managed to provide a healthy and comfortable environment for patients, staff and carers

	Design and construction	Operation and maintenance
1	• Is the HCS designed and built so as to provide comfortable and healthy conditions?	• Are the HCS buildings managed so as to maintain comfortable and healthy conditions?
2	• Is the ventilation of the HCS designed to minimize airborne disease transmission, for example, severe acute respiratory syndrome?	• Is the ventilation of the HCS appropriately managed and health-care workers properly trained?
3	• Is the lighting system of the HCS sufficient to ensure safe working conditions and security, and is it appropriate to local conditions?	• Is the lighting system correctly operated and maintained?
4	• Does the design of the HCS respect national guidance to minimize the spread of contamination (e.g. *Legionella*)?	• Are the HCS activities organized to minimize the spread of contamination?
5	• Is the HCS easily accessible by people with physical handicaps and does it have sufficient space (e.g. between beds) to minimize the spread of contamination?	• Is space in the HCS used in the most effective way for easy access and to minimize the spread of contamination?

HCS, health-care setting

10 Control of vector-borne disease

Patients, staff and carers are protected from disease vectors

	Design and construction	Operation and maintenance
1	• Are HCS environments protected from vector-borne disease?	• Are vector-breeding sites avoided or controlled?
2	• Are HCS buildings designed and built to exclude disease vectors?	• Are inbuilt protective measures effectively used and maintained?
3	• Is insecticide sprayed in and around the HCS?	• Are barriers or repellents used to reduce exposure to vectors?
4	• Are HCSs equipped with bednets and window screens?	• Are all patients, and particularly patients with vector-borne diseases, treated or protected to prevent further transmission?
5	• Are there facilities to safely contain the waste produced?	• Are infectious substances removed or covered or disposed of immediately and completely?

HCS, health-care setting

11 Information and hygiene promotion

Correct use of environmental health facilities is encouraged by hygiene promotion and by management of staff, patients and carers

	Design and construction	Operation and maintenance
1	• Is there a plan for hygiene promotion and staff management?	• Are staff aware of this plan?
2	• Are staff informed about changes and updated about plans or strategies?	• Do staff follow new procedures?
3	• Are staff adequately trained in infection control procedures?	• Do staff follow infection control procedures correctly and consistently?
4	• Is there sufficient communication support available for hygiene information?	• Do staff provide appropriate hygiene information to carers and patients?
5	• Are health-care setting facilities designed so as to be easy to use and maintain hygienically?	• Are health-care setting facilities maintained so as to be easy to use hygienically?

5 Glossary

Autoclave	A device to expose items to steam at a high pressure and temperature to decontaminate the materials or render them sterile. Some autoclaves are used for medical devices; others are used for the treatment of waste.
Coagulation–flocculation	Coagulation is the clumping of particles, which causes impurities to settle to the bottom. It may be induced by coagulants (e.g. lime, aluminium sulfate and iron salts). Flocculation in water and wastewater treatment is the agglomeration or clustering of colloidal and finely-divided suspended matter after coagulation by gentle stirring (by either mechanical or hydraulic means) so the suspended matter can be separated from water or sewage.
Colour comparator (or colour-match comparator)	Equipment used to measure a chemical parameter (e.g. chlorine in water) by adding a specific reagent to the sample and comparing the colour obtained with a colour scale (e.g. DPD for testing chlorine in water).
Disinfection	A process of removing or inactivating microorganisms without complete sterilization.
DPD	A reagent used for determining chlorine in water by colour comparison (abbreviation of N,N-diethyl-p-phenylenediamine).
Environmental surfaces in the context of a health-care setting	Floors, walls, ceilings, table tops, etc.
Health-care associated	An outcome (usually an infection) that occurs in any health-care setting as a result of medical care. The term "health-care associated" replaces "nosocomial", the latter term being limited to adverse infectious outcomes occurring only in hospitals.

Housekeeping surfaces	Environmental surfaces that are not involved in direct delivery of patient care in health-care settings.
Infiltration trench	A shallow trench, containing gravel and a porous pipe, which enables water to percolate into the soil over a larger area, and therefore with a greater infiltration capacity, than a soakaway pit.
Sedimentation	The act or process of depositing sediment from suspension in water. The term also refers to the process whereby solids settle out of wastewater by gravity during treatment.
Soakaway pit or soakpit	A simple excavation in the ground, either lined or filled with stones, that allows water to percolate into the surrounding soil.
Sterilization	The use of a physical or chemical procedure to destroy all microbial life. The most practical method in health-care settings is saturated steam sterilization: exposure to steam saturated with water at 121°C at 1.05 bar for 30 minutes, or 134°C at 2.10 bar for 13 minutes in an autoclave.
Thermotolerant coliform bacteria or faecal coliforms	Bacteria that are used as indicators of faecal contamination of water, for example, as water quality indicators. The bacteria in the coliform group are able to form colonies on selective media at 44°C. Typically, most thermotolerant bacteria are of the species *Escherichia coli*, which is commonly found in faeces.
Turbidity	Cloudiness in water caused by particles in suspension, which makes chemical disinfection of the water less effective. Turbidity is commonly measured in nephelometric turbidity units (NTU) and can be determined visually using simple equipment.

6 Further reading

Centers for Disease Control and Prevention (2003). *Guidelines for environmental infection control in health care facilities*. Recommendations of CDC and the Healthcare Infection Control Practices Advisory Committee (HICPAC). Atlanta, GA (available at http://www.cdc.gov/ncidod/dhqp)

Diaz L, Savage G (2003). *Risks and costs associated with the management of infectious wastes*. Manila, World Health Organization (Western Pacific Regional Office) (available at http://www.wpro.who.int/publications)

Escombe AR et al. (2007). Natural ventilation for the prevention of airborne contagion. *PLoS Medicine*, 4:309–317.

Franceys R, Pickford J, Reed R (1992). *A guide to the development of on-site sanitation*. Geneva, World Health Organization (available at http://wedc.lboro.ac.uk/publications)

Harvey P, Baghri S, Reed R (2002). *Emergency sanitation: assessment and programme design*. Loughborough, UK, Water, Engineering and Development Centre (available at http://wedc.lboro.ac.uk/publications)

Harvey P (2007). *Excreta disposal in emergencies – a field manual*. Loughborough, UK, Water, Engineering and Development Centre (available at http://wedc.lboro.ac.uk/publications/)

Hazel J, Reed R (2005). *Water and sanitation for disabled people and other vulnerable groups — designing services to improve accessibility*. Loughborough, UK, Water, Engineering and Development Centre (available at http://wedc.lboro.ac.uk/publications)

Jensen PA et al. (2005). Guidelines for preventing the transmission of *Mycobacterium tuberculosis* in health care settings, 2005. *MMWR Recommendations and Reports*, 54:1–141.

Médecins Sans Frontières (2005). *Essential water & sanitation requirements for health structures*. Unpublished document. Brussels, MSF.

Pessoa-Silva CL et al. (2004). Healthcare-associated infections among neonates in Brazil. *Infection Control and Hospital Epidemiology*, 25:772–777.

Pittet D (2001). Improving adherence to hand hygiene practice: a multidisciplinary approach. *Emerging Infectious Diseases*, 7(2):234–240 (available at http://www.cdc.gov/ncidod/eid)

Prüss A, Giroult E, Rushbrook P, eds. (1999). *Safe management of wastes from health care activities*. Geneva, World Health Organization (available at http://www.who.int/water_sanitation_health)

Rozendaal JA (1997). *Vector control: methods for use by individuals and communities*. Geneva, World Health Organization (available at http://www.who.int)

Venter SN, September SM (2006). *The effect of water quality on the outcome of hand hygiene*. Department of Microbiology and Plant Pathology, University of Pretoria.

WHO (1993). *Guidelines for cholera control*. Geneva, World Health Organization (available at http://www.who.int/csr/resources/publications/en)

WHO (1997). *Guidelines for drinking-water quality*, 2nd ed. Vol. 3. Surveillance and control of community supplies. Geneva, World Health Organization (available at http://www.who.int/water_sanitation_health/dwq/gdwq2v1/en/index2.html)

WHO (2001). *Five keys to safer food*. Geneva, World Health Organization (Poster WHO/SDE/PHE/FOS/01) (available at http://www.who.int/foodsafety/consumer/en)

WHO (2002a). *Managing water in the home: accelerated health gains from improved water supply*. Geneva, World Health Organization (WHO/SDE/WSH/02.07) (available at http://www.who.int/entity/water_sanitation_health/dwq/wsh0207/en/, see also http://www.who.int/entity/household_water)

WHO (2002b). *Prevention of hospital-acquired infections*. Geneva, World Health Organization. (WHO/CDS/CSR/EPH/2002.12.) (available at http://www.who.int/csr/resources/publications)

WHO (2004a). *Safe health care waste management: policy paper*. Geneva, World Health Organization, (available at http://www.healthcarewaste.org)

WHO (2004b). *Practical guidelines for infection control in health care facilities*. New Delhi/Manila, World Health Organization (South-East Asia Regional Office/Western Pacific Regional Office), (SEARO Regional Publication, No. 41/WPRO Regional Publication) (available at http://www.wpro.who.int/publications)

WHO (2004c). *First adapt then act! A booklet to promote safer food in diverse settings*. New Delhi, World Health Organization (Regional office for South-East Asia) (SEA-EH-546) (available at http://www.who.int/foodsafety/consumer)

WHO (2005a). *Health through safe health care: safe water, basic sanitation and waste management in health care settings*. Geneva, World Health Organization (available at http://www.healthcarewaste.org)

WHO (2005b). *Management of solid health care waste at primary health care centres: a decision-making guide*. Geneva, World Health Organization (available at http://www.who.int/water_sanitation_health/medicalwaste/decisionmguide_rev_oct06.pdf)

WHO (2005c). *World health report 2005*. Geneva, World Health Organization (available at http://www.who.int/whr/2005/en)

WHO (2006). *Guidelines for drinking-water quality incorporating the first addendum to third edition, Volume 1, Recommendations*, (3rd ed.). Geneva, World Health Organisation (available at http://www.who.int/water_sanitation_health/dwq/gdwq3rev/en/index.html)

WHO (2007). *Legionella and the prevention of legionellosis.* Geneva, World Health Organisation (available at http://www.who.int/water_sanitation_health/emerging/legionella/en/index.html)

WHO (advanced draft). *WHO guidelines on hand hygiene in health care.* Geneva, World Health Organization (available at http://www.who.int/patientsafety)

WHO and CDC (Centers for Disease Control and Prevention) (1998). *Infection control for viral haemorrhagic fevers in the African health care setting.* Geneva, World Health Organization (available at http://www.who.int/csr/resources/publications/en)

WHO and FAO (Food and Agriculture Organization) (2007). *How to prepare powdered infant formula in care settings*, Geneva, World Health Organization (available at http://www.who.int/foodsafety/publications/micro/pif_guidelines.pdf)